Vegetarian Diet for Beginners

The Essential Guide to a Healthy and Balanced Plant-Based Eating

Gwenda Flores

Table of Contents

Chapter 1

History of Vegetarianism

To get a good understanding of being a vegetarian, vegetarian food, and cooking it will help to learn about the origins of Vegetarianism. Vegetarianism can be traced back to ancient Egyptian society where many religious sects abstained from eating meat or wearing clothing that was made from animal skins due to their beliefs in reincarnation.

The practice could also be found in ancient Greece. Most notably, famed scholar Pythagoras, known for his contributions in the field of mathematics believed that being a vegetarian was an essential part of being a good human and would help lead to a peaceful existence. The idea of being a vegetarian was hotly debated by the Greeks throughout their civilization. This was one idea that Romans did not share with Greeks. Romans saw animals as a source of food and entertainment for the masses.

Vegetarianism in Religion

Adhering to a vegetarian diet is central to many religions. Buddhism shows kindness to all living things and its believers hold many animals to be scared for what they provide to the humans whether it is milk or as work animals to help plow the fields. Followers of Christianity had different views when it came to being a vegetarian. Christians believe that the humans reign over all other living things on Earth meaning that they believe that animals are here for their use whether that means as beasts of burden or as a food source. However, that does not mean that all Christians are carnivores. Throughout history, different sects of Christians have broken with the mainstream beliefs and preached a vegetarian lifestyle. Vegetarianism played a key role for Christians in Eastern Europe; among these groups were the Bogomils that rose up in the 900's in what is now modern-day Bulgaria. The Bogomils were heretics because they spoke out against what they saw as the excesses of the monasteries and the Eastern Orthodox Church; they rejected the physical world and forswore the consumption of eggs, meat, and cheese that led them to lead a vegetarian lifestyle.

Hinduism

While not all Hindu's practice vegetarianism lifestyle a substantial portion of the followers of religion up to 35 percent adhere to a vegetarian lifestyle. Those that live as vegetarians believe that idea of nonviolence applies to animals and that by avoiding the slaughter of animals, they will not bring bad karma upon their family.

Influence of vegetarianism on the Hindu religion came from its predecessor Brahmanism in which violence against animals was strictly controlled with its scriptures only allowing the slaughter of animals for religious sacrifice.

In Addition, the Brahmanism views are also expressed in Hindu law book the *Dharmaśāstra*, which denounced slaughter of animals and consumption of meat unless it was performed in a proper religious sacrifice performed by priests. Today, the slaughter of animals based on these principles has almost come to an end.

Other Religions

Other major religions throughout the world to include Judaism, Christianity, and Islam have followers that adhere to a vegetarian diet, but the religions do not have a strict policy concerning consumption of animals.

However, when it comes to Judaism and Islam followers of these religions will not consume meat unless it has been slaughtered through the traditional halal method for Muslims and kosher method for followers of Judaism.

While both religions allow their followers to eat the meat that has been prepared in the proper manner, they both avoid eating pork, and meat from the carnivorous animals to include birds of prey.

Chapter 2

Types of Vegetarians

I f you are looking to join the vegetarian lifestyle, there are different options from which you can choose. These different options give you the opportunity to ease your way into the scene without having to jump into the deep end with no life vest. You no longer must make the decision to swear off meat all together to be a vegetarian and you can choose to be one of the four types.

Strict Vegetarian/Vegan

Strict vegetarians are also known as vegans and as their name implies, they do not eat any products that derive from animals, to include cheese, eggs, and cream. Vegans will replace the nutrients that are found in food that comes from animals with different foodstuffs.

For example, vegans use tofu to replace meat that may be found in a dish along with the use of plant cream and plant milk. The nutrients that humans get from eggs and cheeses are replaced with substitution of applesauce and certain ground seeds like flax.

Strict vegetarians also have their own variations of foods that meat eaters consume. If you take the time to visit your local health food store, you have no problem finding vegetarian sausage, vegetarian burgers, vegetarian chicken nuggets, and vegetarian bacon. To replace what nutrition that is lost by not eating meat nutritionists recommend that vegans have a minimum of three servings a day of vegetables that include the dark green and leafy vegetables such as spinach and broccoli, along with vegetables like carrots.

To further their nutritional intake nutritionists, recommend that strict vegetarians also consume at least five servings a day of whole grains like pasta, bread, and rice. To comply with nutritionist guidelines strict vegetarians should also have three servings of fruit and at least two servings of beans, peas, or lentils.

Vegetarian Cooking

There is a different method of cooking for a vegetarian lifestyle. You can also find out the nutritional value in your diet. Many people may not find vegetarian cooking as interesting as the non-vegetarian cooking. There are different methods and styles of preparing vegetarian food as well. All the various means will hence increase your interest in the vegetarian preparation. The simple thought of vegetarian cooking can thus make cooking interesting.

You can find versatility in vegetarian foods. You can also prepare them in several different ways. The best example is to slice up an eggplant into thick portions of about an inch. Then you can make it more creative by layering them with parmesan and ricotta. Special use of mozzarella cheese for vegetarian lasagne is the best example.

Take egg plant and add a small number of breadcrumbs to it and always fry it in olive oil. Olive oil has less fat containing elements and that is good for health as well. Green salad should be consumed because it has great nutritional value.

The level of nutrition you can get from vegetarian food will have the capacity to suffice your requirements. Egg burgers should also be tried as a part of vegetarian diet. The protein part from eggs gives lot of strength to the body.

Usage of spices should be given emphasis because spices can make or break the taste. After the dish is prepared you should try and sprinkle some asparagus to add more taste to the dish. You can try butter spray to get an amazing taste. If you want to experience some tangy twist you can try spritz broccoli which is steamed with a dash of lemon juice to add flavour.

You must think outside the box if you want to do some vegetarian cooking. There are exciting ways to make things interesting. Cooking needs a lot of innovation and great cooks of the world believe that there are ten thousand unique dishes that can be prepared by using all the vegetables available in the world. The treatment of tomato can do wonders. Tomato is an excellent vegetable, and you can experiment many different dishes by using tomatoes. If you like cheese, then you can top the tomato with different kind of cheese to add taste to the preparation. Tomato gives unique and defined taste to any vegetarian dish.

You can innovate several types of dishes by using tomatoes. When you have so many options open by using a single vegetable imagine the range of varieties if you explore more vegetables.

Just utilize your creative instincts and you can create wonders with vegetables. Once you become a vegetarian you will fall in love with the vegetables. Living with fewer options is not advisable because you will get bored of eating same dish again and again. Meatless options can make you forget meat. When you have researched well and explored options then you will encourage vegetarianism.

Cooking vegetarian food is indeed one of the easiest things to learn. Even those who fear boiling water or cooking dishes will find vegetarian food very interesting and easy to prepare. Vegetarian cooking is for everyone. It not only has high nutritional value, but also the vegetarian cooking is easy for everyone.

Deborah Madison, America's top chef just recently came out with his bestseller book 'Vegetarian Cooking for Everyone'. One must not think of it as just another vegetarian cooking book. It has some delicious 800 recipes and vital answers to questions about components and procedures of cooking. One can learn new way to cook some known dishes like Guacamole from the book and even some lesser-known ones like Green Lentils with Roasted Beets and Preserved Lemons, and Cashew Curry.

The review in Amazon quotes that the 124-page chapter on vegetables "the heart of matter" can be taken as reference for any vegetarian culinary skills. One may seek its help in buying vegetables or as a manual. "Madison provides equally inspired recipes and guidance for everything from grains and soy to dairy foods and desserts."

For all its readers it has proved to be a great source book and has ensured a great learning experience. In fact, one of the readers confessed that author is writing recipes for everyday kitchen and this is what attracts readers from all age groups. It is not liked those chef books which the reader or a learner feels difficult to prepare. The 'Vegetarian Cooking for Everyone' is a book for everyone. An average cook can even cook or prepare good dishes reading from it.

For a new learner or beginner this is of great help who can feel his confidence being lifted when he can prepare good vegetarian dishes that taste delicious.

'Vegetarian Cooking for Everyone' has been adjudged as a comprehensive book that is of interest to all, even those who want to seek its help in everyday cooking as well. It has recipes for all starting from starters, sizzlers, snacks breakfast lunch and dinner. The ingredients are simple and can be easily found in one's fridge and pantry and cook something great out of it all which is a huge satisfaction and a source of joy.

Anybody can learn the mastering skills of vegetarian cooking from this book. So, go ahead and enjoy the book!

Vegan Vegetarian

The difference between vegetarian and non-vegetarian is widely understood as the eating habits are distinct and obvious. There is another branch of food eating group commonly known as vegan and the difference between vegetarian and vegan is misunderstood. There is no striking difference between vegan and vegetarian eating habits but still people get confused in categorizing these food eating groups. As a layman you will not be able to understand the difference between vegan and vegetarian. People consider these as same foods eating groups because the similarities are obvious and clear.

People believe what they see, and you often spot a vegetarian eating green fresh salads and few broccolis for all three meals. The fact is different vegans and vegetarians consume foods very differently and their ways are not always similar. Understanding the eating trends of this faction will make things clear. Below are few examples.

People who consume dairy products, eggs, fruits, vegetables are categorized as Lacto-ovo-vegetarian. It is one of the most recurrent and frequent type of lacto-vegetarian diet. There are cases where you find these groups eating fish and consuming poultry products.

Lacto-vegetarian: Their diet includes vegetables, healthy nuts, fruits, grains and dairy products. The only difference is egg consumption which this group avoids.

Vegan: The difference between vegans and vegetarian can be understood by following their food habits. Vegans do not include dairy foodstuffs, eggs or any sort of animal products in their regular diet. Not only have these vegans refrained from sporting or wearing anything which is derived from animal products.

Macrobiotic: There are many reasons to follow a diet group. Diet which is followed on grounds of philosophy and spirituality is known as Macrobiotic diet. Health factors are also considered before selecting this diet.

In this diet food is categorized as negative and positive food. The positive group is ying and negative is yang. There are levels of progression in this type of diet. The elimination of animal products is encouraged at all levels. The highest level eliminates even fruits and vegetables and is confined to brown rice. A normal person will get confused between vegetarian diet and lacto-vegetarian. But for vegans and vegetarian it is easy to follow their lifestyle. It is only when you start to follow a diet regime you come to know positives and negatives. You should support all diet groups and food eating habits as far as it is healthy and keeps you strong.

Low Fat Vegetarian Eating

Everyone knows that once you continue with diet devoid of meat, you are assured of low-fat intake. In this way the article title is a bit oxymoron because vegetable diet is out of fat-based products. A question arises as to why we should give this title low fat vegetarian eating. Since fats are also necessary for the body to function properly, emphasis should be given on natural fat-based products. Eating healthy and keeping your fat levels low can be obtained by vegetarianism as well. When natural fats come into picture you should try and accommodate the right proportion of fat in your diet.

There are many sources of fat-based diets. Fishes have the best fat-based elements known as Omega 3 fatty acids. Such fatty acids give us controlled amount of fat that is required by the human body to stay fit. The problem comes when you decide to be vegan and not a vegetarian because vegans do not eat fish. Whet will be the source of fats? This question keeps hunting people who wants to follow vegan type of food group.

Leaving meats and fishes you can derive fats from other products as well.

Extra virgin olive oil, which is also known as EVOO, has fats that are very good for our system. Low fats are always good and work excellent with vegetarians. You should not take this olive oil in excess if you are vegetarian. Proper proportion should be taken to fulfil the fat requirement of the body. Flax seed and oils from flax seeds should be tried to compensate the fat requirement of vegetarians. Nuts cooked with a good amount of pine nuts are also good source of fats for the vegetarians. Peanuts are suggested by many experts to make your diet complete.

The best food to substitute fats in the body is cheese. In case if you are vegetarian, then it is advisable to make cheese an essential part of your diet plan as you have embraced dairy food items and eggs. Cheese stands to be one of finest suited options for diets rich in fats. People belonging to Wisconsin have a natural tendency to intake cheese. The major aspect to keep in mind is that you must opt for good cheese and add it as an essential item of your vegetarian diet. But, the amount of cheese intake must be checked cautiously, since it tastes good but an overwhelming serving of cheese on regular basis can harm your body.

Vegetarian diet includes low fat intake and consuming a total vegan diet is like naturally eating foods low in fat content. You must check on what kind of food you should eat and what to avoid. To conclude a proper mix of all the nutrients and vitamins will form a healthier and a disease-free system. This will also provide you a slimmer body, healthy lifestyle, and an excellent way of living.

Low Carb Vegetarian

Human bodies need various nutrients to stay fit. Being vegetarian is good, but you need to balance the vitamins and nutrients skilfully. The only thing that should come in your mind is the balance of carbs. Carbs are a great source of energy and that is the only reason to consume carbs in proper proportion. Excess of carbs in a vegetarian diet will trigger fat production in human body. Carbs alter sugar which in turn changes into fat and this creates problem if the quantity of conversion is in excess.

Some foods are rich in carbohydrates like rice, potato, and grains, so if you have plans to low down on carb intake, you should minimize the consumption of such foods.

It is also not advisable to completely cut these foods in your diet as these are good source of carbs. Efforts should be done to curtail the consumption of these food products.

Carbs are also present in flour which also includes the whole wheat flour. You should avoid or minimize eating bread if you are serious about the proper carb's intake. Make sure, that the source of your carbs is appropriate to control the suitable consumption of carbs. Stay away from white bread and eat whole grain bread to compensate the carb requirement of body.

Being vegetarian is good, but you must give up lot of things during the process. The diet should include a lot of fresh and green vegetables.

Selection of oils for preparing the food should also be considered. If you are using olive oil you must use the proper quantity to reach the required level of carb. Also consider steaming and grilling of oil to ensure low carb intake. You have natural vitamins in green and leafy vegetables. Do not consume carbohydrates that will make you gain weight.

Different people have different reasons for changing their lifestyle to a vegetarian one. The most basic reason is losing extra weight. Some people also are really concerned about killing of various animals. A well-balanced diet is the most important criteria behind a vegetarian lifestyle. Excess amount of carbohydrates can change into sugar which can gradually lead to gaining extra weight.

Before you follow a vegetarian diet that is also low in carbohydrate content, you must be very careful in finding the exact amount of carbohydrate present in your diet. If amount of carbs is very low, then it may affect your body and most importantly your health. The most important part of a healthy diet is nutrition.

Low Calorie Vegetarian Recipes

Maybe an individual would have preferred a vegetarian standard of living because they wish to drop weight and require low calorie vegan approach to aid them in their weight loss objectives. The excellent news is that merely by changing over to meat free eating; one would be ingesting low calories.

Unrevealed aspect of preparing healthy vegan recipes is to remove the additional flab that makes meals filling.

Initially, when a person is preparing low-fat vegan recipes, people will want to avoid the use of too much oil. An individual can yet use a superior quality additional virgin olive oil for tastings and salads. EVOO has less caloric value and gives some of the "beneficial fats" that our body need. Discourage fried foods while you are preparing vegetarian recipes which are less in caloric value. Even if one does use the added virgin olive oil for frying, despite this, fried foods characteristically have higher calories, so one should shun fried foods as much as feasible.

Steam the vegetables as an alternative and refrain from boiling them. Boiling will deplete the significant nutrients. Grill vegetables for some change. You can also apply a no calorie or light cooking spray to provide them some wetness or even scatter on a little watery lemon juice.

If one's diet permits them to eat the seafood, boil fish despite frying it. It is advisable to grill the fish since grilling is an immense mode to add taste and distinctiveness to their foods.

Spices are main ingredients that can bring a vast change and provide a low-fat vegetarian recipe that is enjoyable and yummy. A lot of recipes of low-calorie vegetarian dishes can be found online.

An individual can also purchase the vegetarian cookery books with low-fat recipes in them. A more practical and an effortless method for making low calorie vegetarian recipes is to just alter usual recipes by using healthy replacements like diet cheeses or replacing plain yogurt for vinegary cream.

If an individual is creative, they will be amazed to discover that you can discover plenteous healthy vegetarian recipes and able utilize these recipes into one's diet that will balance their weight loss targets.

All a person requires is a little learning into where one can make replacements that will turn high calorie foods into light foods with a small amount of variation and numerous thoughts. Embrace low calorie vegan recipes into your daily diet plan and become conscious that you can consume tasty foods while sustaining your meatless standard of living.

It may possibly seem impractical to imagine initiatives a person should take to study to turn to a vegetarian diet.

Nevertheless, it is not as simple as merely hacking meat out of one's diet? Response to that straightforward issue is.... not actually. People perceive that becoming a vegan requires much more effort, than simply refusing to steak or hamburger. An individual would discover that exploring to become a vegan entails a lot of examination and some serious efforts, so that one can be fit and not devoid their body of something that it essentially requires to function completely in the manner it was intended to.

The most important thing one requires to attempt when turning to a vegan diet is to take it leisurely. If you have been habitual of consuming meat for years now, in that case a laid-back attitude will not make much difference. You will have to make some serious and planned efforts to become a vegan. Begin by slashing meat out of your regular diet gradually. You can cut on meat for some days, then switch over to consuming fish or chicken.

This process can eventually help you in quitting meat permanently as body slowly and progressively gets used change in diet.

If an individual desires to realize how to adopt a lacta-vegetarian diet, then they will also have to do petite exploration into the nutrients that are comprised in different vegetables, so a person can be certain that their body is receiving the essential stuff it requires to be well-built as well as efficient. It must be kept in mind that vitamins like B and C as well as minerals like iron and zinc are essential for the human. Calcium and protein are also vital components of a proportionate diet, so one would wish to know the nutritional value of the food that they are consuming. It is necessary to ensure that the body is provided all the essential nutrients and vitamins that it requires to function efficiently.

Because people are removing meat from their diet, they must ensure that they intake sufficient protein into their body. Protein is crucial for the human body and hence when people are studying how to turn into a vegan, they will desire to get substitute supplies of protein in order that their body can work the manner it was intended to.

It is always hard to accept and undergo changes; likewise altering to a vegetarian diet is not as easy as it may be presumed. So, it is very important to do an in-depth analysis before adapting to a new lifestyle. Sometimes, switching over to meatless diet might be difficult. Therefore, it is better to know the positive and negative effects beforehand, because becoming vegetarian involves a lot more than just cutting on meat.

There are several types of vegetarians like some who prefer eating fish and whereas some who do not. On the other hand, there are people who even do not consume the dairy products including cheese and eggs and live on fruits and vegetables. Switching to vegetarian diet is always a preference. One must also keep in mind nutritional supplements that body would require before you shun cottage cheese and other nutritional foods that provide essential nourishment.

It is better to start off slowly and progress gradually to be a total vegetarian. Though it is hard to believe, the entire body system will go through definite changes, since the body will not be getting something which it is very much habitual of. It is always better to reduce the quantity gradually, instead depriving meat from the routine diet suddenly, replace it by in-taking fish or chicken and then start cutting down consumption gradually turning to be a total vegetarian.

The most important part in turning to a vegetarian style is to know the nutritional contents in the food which would be consumed instead of meat. Generally, those who do not approve of a vegetarian lifestyle, have an assumption that their body would be deprived of vital vitamins and minerals if meat is not added in the diet. Although, there are many who have been successful in switching over to a meatless diet. Such individuals have been able to supply their body with necessary nutrients and hence filling in the lag caused by the meatless diet.

Much research has proved that green vegetables like broccoli, kale and spinach contains enormous amounts of calcium and consumption of these green vegetables would give necessary nutrients to stay healthy. As well, nuts are known to be rich source of protein. Consumption of such vegetarian diets can ensure that one gets enough to have a healthy life with balanced nutrition.

Turning to a vegetarian diet is one of the vital aspects that you can do to make your body feel healthy. And for individuals already converted to a vegan style, must have realized that they feel great and have excessive energy and were able lose weight without starving. So, start thinking on this and make a progress towards a satisfying lifestyle.

Vegan diets are known to be very hale and hearty but eating a reasonable food when an individual is a vegetarian, it usually attracts little additional notice. When a person shuns red meat and animal protein out of their diet, they are shunning out a chief resource of protein which their body requires. It means that eating healthy diet as a vegan will entail adding foods into one's diet that will endow with nutrients commonly found in meat foodstuffs.

By exploring a diet consisting of fruits, vegetables, and whole grains, people can easily avail the vitamins and nutrients they want from vegetarian sources so that their vegetarian way of life is healthy and in proportion. By consuming food items like legumes, soy foods, nuts, and eggs, one can obtain the essential protein content that they require to nurture.

One must also keep in mind that other nutrients like the minerals iron, calcium, and the vitamins D and B12, are equally vital for vegans.

Whereas it is factual that removing meat out of one's diet and consuming a diet rich in vegetables, fruits, and grains is healthy. But vegetarians require worrying about other things essential nutrients like receiving the right balance of vitamins and minerals from their diet. Many can constantly take a vitamin add-on, but since a lot of these supplements include animal derivatives, many devoted vegetarians hesitate in taking them. It is essential that one must look out for a diet which is rich in vitamins B and C, iron, and niacin since they are also vital part of a healthy lacto-vegetarian way of life.

A person does not have to forgo one's health when they prefer to become a vegan. Ingestion of healthy vegetarian diet is not an easy task. One must exclusively take leisure time to study and find food items that include nutrients most essential for the body. For this, perhaps you will have to go extensively through several books, magazines or even surf internet.

People can make all kinds of swaps in their diet that can replace meat when are not eating any longer. For instance, one can opt for soy milk as an alternative to cow's milk which in turn will provide the necessary calcium to the body. Including nuts and grains into a vegetarian diet suitably turns it into a healthy diet. Also, nuts and grains are full of proteins which are helpful in developing healthy bones.

Several Studies have revealed that vegetarians generally have healthy eating routine that leads to a fit and healthy body.

They also have a higher tendency to remain healthy and energetic. The thing people need to keep in mind for healthy vegan diet is that they must give particular interest to nutrient content present in the foods that they eat and be sure to eat balanced diet.

Cooking Gourmet Vegetarian

For individuals who are vegan and are fond of cooking gourmand dishes, there are enormous opportunities to explore and find.

There are a huge number of epicurean vegan recipes that an individual can cook in varied places and situations; you just need to seek prospects to do so. Regrettably, space limitation prevents us from enumerating a complete cookbook in this small article. But there are a few recommendations to offer regarding to tasty vegetarian food preparation.

Initially we begin by defining an epicure meal. Now the question arises that is this feasible? A gourmand meal is special meal devoid of meat or spaghetti and it includes converting interesting and rare elements into a masterpiece dishes that are not only delicious but also remarkable in appearance. Evidently, gourmet can be explained by many people in many various ways but cooking a gourmet vegan food entails enough talent. It requires one to put a lot of flavour and ability to convert simple ingredients to artistic creations.

So, what must an individual know to cook a gourmand vegetarian meal? If they have been a lacto-vegetarian for rather some time, they might want to refer to ideas about what one likes to consume and how one can induce innovativeness to make it unusual and delicious as well as mouth-watering.

If people are novel to vegetarian style of cooking, the best process is to bear in mind the type of gourmet meals they have had before. It is very true that almost each one of us has had vegetarian meals. One must always look out for ways one can shut out the meat portion in the dish, while still maintaining intact the essence. With a little mind and resourcefulness, this can be made possible - we know almost all can!

An individual can find enormous and diverse recipe books that are out-and-out devoted to gourmand vegetarian style of cooking in their local bookstore, on several web sites, and online. Surf for cooking methods that contain constituents that fascinate all and then try the recipe. Many will not be able to cook a gourmet vegetarian feast if they start from anywhere. But by stringently following the instructions, you can avert a gastronomic failure.

Cooking a gastronome meal can be a real adventurous and rejuvenating thing that a person ever does as a vegan chef. A lot of people believe the vegetarian way of life comprises of perplexity and inquisitiveness.

When one can easily demonstrate that catering a vegetarian banquet that is epicurean, striking, and yummy, they may just wave them toward their side of the boundary.

But do not struggle very hard. Being a lacto-vegetarian is not for one and all. The finest things people can do is to cook with their heart and stay proper to their dedication of living a vegetarian style of living which signifies cooking foodie meals that savour like they have mutton when they do not have any meat content.

Health Benefits

Research studies have shown that people that adhere to a strict vegetarian diet and follow the recommended nutritional servings have a lower risk of cardiovascular disease as well as lower levels of obesity. Studies have also shown that a properly executed vegetarian diet is safe for all ages of human life, along with situations that put more nutritional needs on the body such as pregnancy.

On the other hand, if a strict vegetarian does not follow a properly planned diet, they may suffer from shortages of vitamin B12, Omega-3 fatty acids, vitamin D, iron, zinc, among other vital vitamins and minerals.

To counter act some of the deficiencies that can occur with being a strict vegetarian it is recommended vegetarians eat foods that are rich in vitamin B12 or take a vitamin B12 supplement to ensure that blood levels maintain their normal levels. The reason for this is that vitamin B12 is essential to the formation of new red blood cells, DNA synthesis, and proper nerve function. By not consuming the recommended dosage of vitamin B12, strict vegetarians are at risk for a variety of health problems to include anaemia.

This is especially critical in strict vegetarians that become pregnant. Vegetarian women should supplement their diet with B12. Low levels of B12 when breastfeeding have been linked to neurological problems in children. It is also important during pregnancy for a strict vegetarian to ensure that they follow the recommended daily servings because consuming a vegetarian diet has been linked to low birth weights in new-borns.

Lacto-vegetarian

The Lacto-vegetarians follow most of dietary recommendations of strict vegetarians except that they consume milk, cheese, yogurt, and butter but not eggs. This type of vegetarian diet is popular in India. Lacto-vegetarianism is in keeping with the Eastern religions such as Hinduism, Sikhism, and Buddhism and their belief in non-violence. Hindu's believe that you are affected by the type of food that you consume and being a lacto-vegetarian helps them maintain an inner peace by not consuming the flesh of any animals.

Health Benefits

This type of vegetarian diet is good for people that want to keep their cholesterol levels at an acceptable number. They can do this because lacto-vegetarians abstain from eating fish and egg yolks that are high in cholesterol. Just like strict vegetarians, those who choose to become lacto-vegetarians should maintain a proper diet with the recommended servings of vegetables, legumes, whole grains, and fruits.

They should also back up their food selections with vitamin supplements such as B12, iodine, and choline.

Furthermore, while vegetarian diets have been deemed healthy for all ages, pregnant women should ensure that they are getting all the recommended nutrition. If they do not, they are putting their new-born at risk for low birth weight, neurological disorders, and vision problems.

They can help avoid these problems by taking the vitamins and minerals along with DHA supplements to help the development of the new-borns vision.

Lacto-Ovovegetarian

A person who chooses to become a lacto-ovovegetarian is a vegetarian who does not eat meat but does consume dairy products and eggs. This type of vegetarian diet is more common in Western culture. This is also the most common type of vegetarianism that is catered to in mainstream restaurants. This means that if you are going to go to dinner with someone who is a lacto-ovovegetarian you do not have to look for a restaurant that caters exclusively to vegetarians because most restaurants will have vegetarian options available on their menu.

This type of vegetarian lifestyle is popular with Seventh Day Adventists. The Seventh Day Adventist church recommends that its followers eat a diet that is rich in whole grain bread, cereal, and pasta. It also calls for the liberal use of green leafy vegetables and fruits along with a modest number of nuts, beans, and seeds. When it comes to consuming dairy products Seventh Day Adventists advises its followers to choose the low-fat varieties of milk, yogurt, and cheese and does allow for the consumption of eggs.

Health Benefits

Like other types of vegetarianism, being a lacto-ovovegetarian has healthy benefits. Lacto-ovovegetarian usually consume a diet that is lower in saturated fats and cholesterol than the traditional diets that include the consumption of meat, which can aid in reducing the risk of atherosclerosis and lowering blood pressure.

Some people who suffer from diabetes can better control their blood glucose levels through implementation of a vegetarian diet. This is possible through the consumption of vegetarian foods such as legumes, fruit, and green leafy vegetables that can make your body more responsive to insulin. In addition, the vegetarian diet is low in fat and high in fiber, which in turn can help you maintain a healthy weight further controlling blood glucose levels.

Moreover, as well as being helpful for people who suffer from diabetes, a vegetarian diet has also been shown to lower a person's risk for cancer. The vegetarian foods are rich of antioxidants and phytochemicals, which have been shown to lower the risk of cancer. To that end, consuming meat has been shown to increase a person's chance of getting prostate and colon cancer. Additionally, studies have shown that diets high in fat have been linked to a higher risk of breast cancer.

Flexitarian

The term "flexitarian" is relatively new and is used to describe people who follow a vegetarian diet for the most part but will occasionally eat meat. You might meet people who call themselves semi-vegetarian - is the same as being a flexitarian. This might be a good option for someone who is making the transition from being a meat eater to a vegetarian. You can try to avoid eating meat, but if you want to have a small break, it is okay, and you will not feel like you have failed. One compromise that some flexitarians do when eating meat is that when they eat meat, they only eat animals have been raised organically or free range.

Being a flexitarian has become somewhat of an argument in the vegetarian culture. Some vegetarians feel any consumption of any meat products is strictly forbidden, while others have embraced the idea that any reduction in people consuming animals is a positive. The benefit of being a flexitarian is that you can get essential protein through meat and will be less prone to need outside supplements to maintain healthy levels of vitamins and minerals.

Chapter 3

The United States

In a recent study that was performed, it was determined that just over three percent of Americans are vegetarian or approximately nine million people. Three million of those who claimed to be vegetarian identified themselves as vegan meaning that they do not eat any products that come from animals to include dairy products and eggs. Additionally, nearly ten percent of U.S. adults or thirty million stated that they follow a mostly vegetarian diet.

Most adults that stated that they follow a vegetarian diet were female at sixty percent with males at forty percent. There was also a slight majority for people aged eighteen to thirty-four suggesting that the decision to become a vegetarian is one that takes place early in life. The main reason for deciding to become a vegetarian was health concerns, with over fifty percent giving that reason.

Origins

Vegetarianism in the United States was endorsed by the American Health Convention in 1838. However, vegetarians remained somewhat of an enigma in American society with only one percent of the population adhering to a vegetarian diet up until 1971. This percentage has tripled over the last forty years with now over 3% of Americans following a vegetarian diet. This number is only sure to grow as vegetarian parents introduce their children to the lifestyle. There are some scholars that point to the year 1971 as the birth of vegetarianism in the United States due to the release of the book *Diet for a Small Planet* by Francis Moore Lappé.

Important Literary Contributions

In *Diet for a Small Planet*, Lappé makes the case for conserving food after she learned that it takes fourteen times the amount of grain to feed an animal compared to the amount of meat that can be consumed from the same animal. In fact, she determined that livestock consume about eighty percent of all the grain that is produced in the United States, which takes it out of the mouths it could feed at a much lower price than animal meat can.

The early 1970's also saw the popularity of soybeans grow in the United States. The main credit for this can be traced to a vegetarian commune farm in Tennessee that was given the unimaginative title "The Farm". The soybean-based product tofu was brought to the attention of mainstream America through the publication of *The Farm Cookbook*.

As the twentieth century wore on more books were being published about being a vegetarian. In 1987, John Robbins published the book *Diet for a New America,* which built upon studies that had been done on vegetarian diets along with adding new information and it presented the information in an objective manner. One of the main points that *Diet for a New America* made was the contrast between the health benefits of being a vegetarian to how eating a meat-based diet could lead to a higher incidence of medical problems such as hypertension, cardiovascular disease, and some cancers.

Trend of publishing new findings in health and vegetarianism continued into the 1990's, which saw the publication of *Dr. Dean Ornish's Program for Reversing Heart Disease* in 1990. In this publication, Dr. Ornish showed through his research how heart disease could be reversed through the implementation of a mostly vegetarian, low fat diet. It was during the 1990's that the American Dietetic Association began to espouse benefits of a vegetarian diet for its benefits in health, help with lowering blood glucose levels in people who suffer from diabetes.

England

Vegetarianism in England has a long and distinctive history. Even before the term "vegetarian" was coined there where people in the church that advocated a diet that was free of animal flesh. One of the first church officials to champion a diet free of meat was the leader of the Bible Christian Church, Reverend William Cowherd.

To Reverend Cowherd, consumption of animal flesh was not in keeping with the natural order of the world and could lead to aggression.

The idea that following a vegetarian diet was morally virtuous caught on in England. This can be seen with formation of the Vegetarian Society on September 30, 1847 in Ramsgate, Kent. The society immediately had over one hundred people sign up to be members, a number that rose to over two hundred and fifty the following year. The idea of vegetarianism spread quickly across the country and by 1849, the Vegetarian Society newsletter *The Vegetarian Messenger* had a circulation of approximately five thousand.

Expansion

Vegetarianism in England spread relatively fast, 1877 saw the formation of The London Food Reform Society, which not only swore off animal flesh but alcohol and tobacco.

Vegetarian meetings were held all across Britain, from Glasgow to London and Liverpool, the movement became so influential that even a vegetarian hotel was opened in Birmingham at the turn of the twentieth century.

Throughout twentieth-century vegetarianism continued to grow throughout England, with interruptions to vegetarian diets due to the First and Second World Wars. It was after the Second World War, in the 1950's, that vegetarianism in England began to prosper once again.

Restaurants in London started in include vegetarian selections, which not only attracted vegetarians to their restaurants but also gave customers the opportunity to try something new. Restaurants offering vegetarian options on their menus coincided with vegetarian societies and clubs across the country beginning to work together and putting out a common message about the benefits of living a vegetarian lifestyle.

As in the United States, medical professionals, doctors, and researchers became involved in investigating vegetarian diet. Prior to Dr. Dean Ornish in the United States, Dr. Frank Wokes studied the vegetarian diet in England starting in the 1950's. His research, like Dr. Ornish's that was to follow showed the benefits of eating a vegetarian diet and its help with weight loss and lowering the risk of cardiac problems in people that ate a vegetarian based diet. Today, vegetarian restaurants can be found across England.

India

Perhaps no other country on the planet is as closely associated with vegetarian cuisine than India. Indians have been closely linked with vegetarianism dating back to the birth of Buddhism and its emphasis on non-violence. Their belief in non-violence goes hand in hand with its reverence for cows and seeing them as an animal that provides for them so its flesh should not be consumed by humans.

That is not to say that all Indians are vegetarian, but it does enjoy popularity in many of India's states. Many Indian states have populations that are over fifty percent vegetarian with more states just below that level, in a country that has over a billion people; it makes for a lot of vegetarians. The state that boasts the largest percent, nearly seventy percent vegetarian is Gujarat located on the western coast of India.

Gujarat

Their morning meal is usually made up of rice, lentils, roti, and vegetables, in the evening a favourite meal is known as khichdi kadhi, which is a dish made up of rice and lentils. However, their food selections are not just limited to rice and lentils. Staples of Gujarati's cuisine include cereal, buttermilk, fruits, vegetables, yogurt, chutney, ghee, and pickles along with various spices that are used during food preparation.

Andhra Pradesh

The southern state of Andhra Pradesh is also well known for its vegetarian dishes. Andhra Pradesh cuisine is infused with the use of different varieties of pickles that are available at different times of the year. It is also known for its spiciness, which is why you will find curd served quite often with meals as a counterbalance. Like the cuisine that is found in Gujarat, food staples in Andhra Pradesh are rice, lentils, and various vegetables.

Punjab

The Punjab region of India is known for its diversity in food preparation, this includes many vegetarian dishes. Punjabi cuisine incorporates the use of ghee, or clarified butter, along with rice cooked in sugar cane juice. Most of the dishes include whole wheat with the use of garlic and ginger for seasoning. Like other regions and states in India, you will find dishes that have lentils and are served with curd to take a bite out of the spiciness. You will also find dishes that are prepared using buttermilk as well as the use of red and black beans.

Germany

At first thought, one might not think of Germany as having a sizable vegetarian population, especially with it being famous for its sausage and schnitzel. However, recent studies have shown that Germany's population is about eleven percent vegetarian, which is a greater percent of the population being vegetarian than even the United States. Some of this growth in vegetarianism is Germany can be traced to its increasing population diversity. According to new government data, nearly one in five Germans has immigrated to Germany. This growing diversity had added to the variety of foods that are available at

German supermarkets as well as adding to the assortment of restaurants that cater to immigrants and native Germans.

Shopping for vegetarian foods in Germany can be a little tricky if you are not familiar with the language or have a native German to help you pick the right packages. This is because unlike countries such as the United States and England, Germany does not have system to label their food as vegetarian. So if you find yourself in this predicament get a good German dictionary so you will be able to make out what the ingredients are in the package of food that you what to buy.

If you choose to take your meals at a restaurant, you should not have any trouble finding vegetarian selections on the menu. This is especially true if you are visiting any of the large cities across the country. However, even the smaller eateries in rural parts of the country have at least one selection available on their menu.

Chapter 4

Vegetarian Food and Your Health

S witching to a vegetarian diet can be an exciting and fun way to attain a healthier lifestyle. As we have previously learned, vegetarians do not eat fish, meat, or poultry. Although some do eat dairy or eggs. If you choose to follow one of these diets and lifestyles, you will find that your risks of contracting certain diseases will fall.

Cardiovascular Disease

Studies that have been conducted on vegetarians have shown that they have lower cholesterol levels that people who consume red meat. This is because cholesterol is found in animal products to include milk and eggs. Therefore, even if you choose to become a lacto-vegetarian you will be consuming much lower levels of cholesterol than if you stayed on a meat-based diet.

To that end, vegetarian meals are also low in saturated fat, one of the leading causes of cardiovascular disease.

In addition, studies have shown that consuming plant proteins instead of animal proteins have led to vegetarians having lower cholesterol levels.

Hypertension

There have also been many studies conducted on vegetarians in concern to their blood pressure. Results have shown that vegetarians, on average, have lower blood pressure than the people who consume red meat as a regular part of their diet.

Adhering to a vegetarian diet is beneficial for people who suffer from hypertension due to it being low in sodium and cholesterol.

In some cases, people who have suffered from hypertension and switched to a vegetarian diet have been able to stop taking medication to keep their blood pressure under control.

Diabetes

Becoming a vegetarian can also be advantageous to people who suffer from diabetes. A vegetarian diet is high in complex carbohydrates and low in fat, which are essential in keeping a diabetic person's blood glucose level at a more normal range.

Some people who suffer from diabetes have been able to come off their medication once they switched to a vegetarian diet, while others have seen a decrease in the amount of self-injected insulin, they require to keep their blood glucose level within an acceptable range.

Cancer

Committing to a vegetarian diet can also reduce the risk of some cancers. Studies have shown that people who live in countries and cultures that have a vegetarian diet or nearly vegetarian diet have a less incidence of breast and colon cancer in their population. It is believed that this is achieved because vegetarian diets are low in fat and high in fiber.

In addition, vegetables are high in beta-carotene that has been shown to help lower the risk of getting cancer. It has also been discovered that people who follow a vegetarian diet have more of what are called killer cells that are able to protect the body by fighting off and killing cells that are turning cancerous.

Other Diseases

Just as vegetarians are at a lower risk of getting some cancers, cardiovascular disease, and diabetes, they are at a lower risk for being afflicted with gallstones, kidney stones, or osteoporosis. This is due to consuming plant proteins instead of animal protein. Eating high quantities of animal protein has been shown in studies to dramatically decrease the amount of calcium from human bones.

With vegetarian diet, the consumption of plant proteins can help people from getting osteoporosis.

Chapter 5

How to Plan a Vegetarian Diet

I f you are making the switch to a vegetarian diet do not be overwhelmed when it comes to making a shopping list so you can start preparing vegetarian meals at home. It is not a difficult job to make sure that you have everything you need to succeed in your new endeavour.

Make sure you buy plenty of grains, green leafy vegetables, beans, and nuts. If you are unsure of how to prepare vegetarian meals, invest in a vegetarian cookbook, which are plentiful at your local bookstore or look online for recipe ideas.

Simple Guidelines for the Beginner

Start with simple and easy to prepare meals such as brown rice and mix in your favourite vegetables, you can even add flavour to rice by adding apple juice to the water when cooking it. Take a trip to your local ethnic market, many of these markets especially ones that cater to people from the Middle East will have a variety of vegetarian selections available and will be able to give you some pointers about how to prepare food that you might not be familiar with.

To curb your temptations to fall off vegetarian wagon while you have a day out, pack some nuts, granola, fresh or dried fruit, along with some juice.

Chapter 6

What about Protein?

Getting the right amount of protein is important to maintain human health. It was once believed that a vegetarian diet could not deliver the proper amount of protein that humans needed without including at least some red meat. However, this has been proven not to be the case. If you follow a proper vegetarian diet with the right amount of bean, grains, lentils, and vegetables you get all essential amino acids that you need to maintain a healthy diet.

The benefit of consuming plant proteins instead of animal protein is that you will not only eating a healthier diet but your risk for many medical problems will be lowered.

Eating a diet that is high in animal protein increases your risk for developing the kidney disease, certain cancers, kidney stones, and even osteoporosis.

How about Calcium?

Do not be worried that by becoming a vegetarian that you will be not getting the required amount of calcium that is needed to maintain your body's health. The benefit of being a vegetarian is that a proper vegetarian diet does not contain protein from animals. Diets that are high in animal proteins have been shown to cause bones to lose calcium and possibly lead to osteoporosis.

Along with the use of plant proteins to maintain healthy calcium levels vegetarians can find foods that are a good source of calcium. Good sources of calcium in a vegetarian diet include soymilk, soybeans, lentils, almonds, and some dried fruit.

Chapter 7

Supermarket Shopping Tips

When you have made the decision to become a vegetarian you will also have task of relearning your favourite supermarket. You will have to find things on aisles that you may have never been down before. As most supermarkets are generally laid out in like fashion, it is good to know the sections where vegetarian foods can be found.

Most supermarkets now offer a health food section, and it is here where you will find products like vegetarian burgers, sausage, and roasts. Refrigerated section of your supermarket is where you will find vegetarian hotdogs, tofu, vegetarian bacon, hummus, and egg-free pasta. Other vegetarian staples will be where they have always been, these items include rice, beans, pasta, spaghetti sauce. Of course, you should already know where they keep vegetables at your local supermarket.

A Sample of a Vegetarian Menu

Making switch to become a vegetarian does not mean that your daily meals will be filled with bland food that resembles bark from a tree. There are many choices that you can make to have delicious and attractive looking meals. For breakfast, have oatmeal, toast with peanut butter, your favourite fruit, and cereal with soymilk and top it off with a sliced banana or your other favourite fruit. At lunchtime, you can choose from having a veggie burger, garden salad, baked sweet or regular potato topped with your favourite vegetable, hummus, or a hearty vegetable soup with crackers, or a bowl of fresh fruit. For dinner, you could choose from having burritos stuffed with beans, rice, tomatoes, and avocado, or a fresh garden salad. You could opt for a Chinese stir-fry made with tofu and vegetables such as broccoli, onions, and ginger or vegetarian sausage. You could also have pasta topped with a vegetarian spaghetti sauce or your favourite vegetables with a nice vegetarian dip. If you get hungry during day, make sure that you have some vegetarian snacks on hand like fresh fruit, trail mix, dried fruit, or a soy-based yogurt.

Chapter 8

Forget about the Five Food Groups

Most of us can remember way back in school learning about the five food groups and what the recommended servings were from each group, but the five food groups that we learned about are no more. What was once five groups have now been pared down to four. This new and improved four food groups was developed in 1991 to try to reduce the amount of cholesterol and fats that adults were consuming with the previous five-food group plan.

Group 1 – Vegetables

It is now recommended that adults consume at least five servings of vegetables every day. While it was already known that vegetables are good for you, the more that is learned about the healthy properties in vegetables the more they should be incorporated into your daily routine.

Vegetables are rich in vitamin C, iron, calcium, beta-carotene, and riboflavin. Vegetables that are of the dark green and leafy variety like broccoli and spinach are full of these nutrients. Vegetables that are yellow or orange such as carrots, squash, sweet potatoes, pumpkins have even more nutrients like beta-carotene than green leafy vegetables. For vegetables, the serving size is either 1-cup of raw vegetables or ½ cup of cooked vegetables.

Group 2 – Whole Grains

For whole grains, it is recommended that adults should have at least three servings a day. Whole grains are rich in protein, fiber, B vitamins, and complex carbohydrates. To get the nutrition you need from whole grains you need to know what foods to choose. Foods that are considered whole grain include cereal, tacos, whole grain bread, whole grain pasta, and corn. Serving sizes for whole grains are as follows, ½ cup of rice or pasta, ½ cup of cereal, or one slice of bread.

Group 3 – Fruit

When it comes to fruit, it is recommended that adults should have at least three servings a day. Eating fresh fruit is important because it is rich in beta-carotene and vitamin C. It is important that at least one of the serving of fruit that you incorporate into your diet should be of the citrus variety such as oranges, strawberries, melon, or peaches. This is because they are full of vit C. Serving sizes for fruit group breakdown like this, ½ cup of cooked fruit, ½ cup of juice, or one medium piece of fruit.

Group 4 – Legumes

It is now recommended that to ensure that you are following a healthy diet you should have at least two servings of legumes every day. Consuming legumes are important for vegetarians: they are good sources of iron, fiber, B vit, protein, calcium, and zinc. Other foods that are considered part of the legume group include chickpeas, refried beans, and tofu.

Chapter 9

Pregnancy and Vegetarianism

When a woman becomes pregnant, her body needs more nutrition in order to help the development of her unborn child. For women that are vegetarian, it does not mean that you must give up being one to ensure you are getting the proper nutrition for yourself and your baby.

What you must do is alter the servings of the four food groups to maximize your nutrition. The good news is that because you we are vegetarian before you became pregnant that you are probably in good health, which is very important for the initial stages of your pregnancy.

Calcium

During pregnancy, it is important to maintain proper nutrition and one of the most important nutrients during pregnancy is calcium. When pregnant, vegetarians should try to have at least four servings of foods that are high in calcium. Foods that are good sources of calcium especially when pregnant include green leafy vegetables, cereals and soymilk that has been fortified with calcium, bok choy, and beans.

Vitamin B12

One vitamin that is lacking in the vegetarian diet is vitamin B12. When a woman is pregnant it is more important than ever to make sure that she is getting all the vitamins she needs to ensure proper development of her unborn child. There are not many food choices for vegetarians to choose from that are good sources of vitamin B12. The best source of vitamin B12 for vegetarians is soymilk that has had vitamin B12 added to it. To ensure that pregnant vegetarian women get right amount of vitamin B12 in their diet it is recommended that they take a B12 supplement. It is important to check label of prenatal vitamins to ensure that vitamin B12 is included in its recommended daily dosage.

Iron

For vegetarians, making sure that they have enough iron in their diet when pregnant should not be a problem. Green leafy vegetables, nuts, beans, and whole grains are all good sources of iron and are staples of the vegetarian diet. To help absorb iron, it is a good idea to eat citrus fruit or drink some juice that has high levels of vitamin C and this will help make sure that pregnant vegetarian women are getting enough iron. Just remember that as pregnancy progresses more iron is needed, so a supplement may be needed.

Protein

During pregnancy, the body's need for protein increases just like many other nutrients. This is another one of advantages of being a vegetarian. The vegetarian diet is full of good sources of protein, soy, whole grains, and legumes are full of protein and if you have been following a proper vegetarian diet, you are probably already getting enough protein during pregnancy.

Suggestions for Meals during Pregnancy

As you have read, when pregnant it is important to maintain a healthy diet and increase the intake of some foods to ensure that the proper amount of nutrients is consumed. To do this, make sure your meals include green leafy vegetables, whole grains, beans, nuts, and fruit. For example, for breakfast have juice, cereal topped with your favourite fruit, or perhaps toast with peanut butter. For lunch, have a healthy garden salad with a nice assortment of fresh fruit. For dinner, have some lentil soup and do not be afraid to add your favourite vegetables to the soup, perhaps broccoli or spinach. For snacks during the day, have some dried fruit, trail mix, or nuts.

Do not forget to include some soymilk that has been fortified with vitamin B12 and take any supplements that have been prescribed. If the decision to breastfeed is made, then the same diet was followed during pregnancy should be continued until the decision is made to stop breastfeeding.

Chapter 10

Vegetarianism and Children

One of the most important things you can do as a parent is to teach your children how to eat healthy. The best way to do this is to start as soon as they are born to set a solid foundation for the rest of their lives. When it comes to new-borns and the decision has been made not to breastfeed use a soy-based formula to ensure that the new-born gets all the necessary nutrients. Do not just use regular soymilk because a new-born needs all the nutrients that the soy-based formula has been fortified with. Do not keep your new-born indoors all the time, make sure that you go out for walks or outing so the new-born can get vitamin D from the sun.

As Your New-born Grows

When your new-born reaches four to five months, it is okay to start introducing them to other foods. Start by offering them pureed fruit like bananas, peaches, or applesauce. You can even try single grain cereal mixed with a little soymilk. Make sure when you introduce new foods to your new-born that you watch closely for any allergic reactions that may occur.

By the time your new-born reaches six months old, they should be ready for vegetables. Make sure that they have been fully cooked and pureed. Good choices to introduce at this time are pureed sweet potatoes, green beans, and carrots. By time your new-born reaches eight months old, you can introduce them to crackers and bread. Their rapid development will continue to astound you and by the time they reach a year old they should be getting nourishment from all four food groups and now is a good time to introduce them to soymilk that has been fortified with vitamin B12. These ages are a guideline to follow, do not be worried if your child does not want fruit at four months or vegetables at six months because all children develop at different rates and when your new-born is ready you will be sure to know it.

Older Children

If you decide to wait until your children get older to introduce them to a vegetarian lifestyle there are some steps that you can follow to make the transition easier for you and your children. Do not try to convert your children overnight into being vegetarians. Start by slowly removing meat from their diet. You can still let them have some of their favourite foods, pizza, for example but instead of topping it with pepperoni or sausage, choose green peppers, onions, or a combination of vegetables. To replace the protein that will be lost by not eating red meat, introduce more beans into their diets, which are a good source of protein.

Do not Rely on Gimmicks

One of the things that parents do when they are changing their children from omnivores to vegetarian is to smother their food with cheese. As you have already read, some vegetarians consume dairy products, so it is not cheating but it is not a great idea to rely on this too much. While cheese can be a nutritious part of a vegetarian diet, it is also high in saturated fat and has a lot of sodium in it, which can be harmful to your child's diet and thus undoing the good that you are trying to do with a vegetarian diet.

Children are Different than Adults

It is important for parents to remember that children are not small adults. There nutritional needs are different from what adults need. Serving children vegetarian foods that are high in fiber is not a good idea because children cannot digest fiber as well as an adult can. In addition, children have smaller stomachs than adults do, so when you are changing their diet to vegetarian, they might need to eat more than three times a day. If you find this is the case with your children try to serve them smaller more frequent meals to ensure they get all the recommended daily servings of the four food groups.

Important Nutrients for Children

A child's body is a living breathing machine and for it to function and grow properly it needs the proper fuel to make it happen. It is the job of the parent to make sure that their diet contains the appropriate amounts of green leafy vegetables, legumes, whole grain, and fruit. By doing this the parent will ensure that their child will get all the necessary iron, calcium, protein, and zinc. Parents also need to be proactive and make sure their children do not sit in front of the television playing video games or Facebooking and get outside to soak in some vitamin D.

Vegetarian children will probably also need to take a vitamin B12 supplement to meet their body's requirement for growth.

Chapter 11

Helpful Tips for Parents

School Lunch

When changing your children's diet parents are bound to come across some obstacles. One of these for parents of school age children is the school lunch. Children that are changing to a vegetarian diet are bound to face some peer pressure from their friends who find it either weird or strange to be a vegetarian. It is important for parents to sit down with their children, explain what benefits of being a vegetarian diet are.

Packing a lunch, with input of the child, can help avoid any slips away from a vegetarian diet. Parents can make sandwiches with hummus with tomatoes or avocado. Peanut butter sandwiches and pretzels are an easy alternative to lunchmeat.

Parents can send a hearty vegetable soup or stew in a thermos as well as leftover pasta with a vegetarian spaghetti sauce. For something on the side send raw vegetables with a vegetarian dip, whole grain muffins, soy-based yogurt, or fresh fruit.

Having Friends Over

One challenge that parents of vegetarian children will face is what to do when their friends come over to play, birthday party, or another event. However, do not fret parents; there are many options available from which to choose that will make you, your children, and their friends happy. Vegetarian hamburgers are widely available at supermarkets and you can include everyone by allowing them opportunity to choose their own condiments, whether that is just ketchup and mustard or avocado, lettuce, onions, tomatoes. Additionally, vegetarian hotdogs are widely available at your local supermarket and unless you know that it is vegetarian, the taste is just about indistinguishable from meat variety. Pizza is another good standby to choose, just make sure that toppings are vegetarian instead of meat. Fruit smoothies are a refreshing treat that not only fun but also healthy.

Family Members

Just because you are part of greater family is vegetarian does not mean that rest of your family is or is knowledgeable about the vegetarian lifestyle. To help your child stay on right track, do not beat around the bush with family members and with parents of your child's friends. Being upfront with them will ensure that they know where you stand and there will not be any misunderstandings when it comes to your child visiting friends and family. To help make things easier when your child visits friends and family send along a dish with them to avoid putting any undue burden on anyone.

Plan Ahead

With most households now either having to have both parents work or headed up by a single parent time is of the essence, so it is important to plan. Get some cookbooks that have recipes for quick, nutritious meals. You can have a cook day, include your children, and make several meals that you can freeze and use throughout the week. This is a great way to get your children involved in the vegetarian lifestyle and a great way to learn what they really like and what they would rather not eat.

Advantages of being a Child Vegetarian

Getting a jump start on a healthy lifestyle by becoming a vegetarian at an early age will benefit children as they grow into adulthood. With childhood obesity becoming more and more of a problem in society being a vegetarian dramatically decrease the chances of that happening. Being a vegetarian early in life will also lessen risk of developing cardiovascular disease, some forms of cancer, and lower chance of suffering a heart attack or stroke. In addition, in some studies vegetarian girls have been shown to start menstruating at a later age than girls who are omnivores, by starting their menarche at a later age studies have shown that it decreases the risk of breast cancer. Along the health benefits of turning to a vegetarian diet at a young age, studies have shown that vegetarian diet may boost brain function.

Chapter 12

Vegetarianism and the Elderly

The elderly population is turning to vegetarianism in greater numbers in recent years. For people who have been omnivores for most of their lives it is important for them to change their diet gradually so not to shock their body. For the elderly it is important for them to see a physician before they make any drastic dietary changes to ensure that they are healthy enough to take on something new. As people grow older, dairy products are less tolerated and meat becomes harder for the elderly to digest. This is one reason why you are never too old to switch to a vegetarian diet. Vegetables, legumes, and fruit are easier to digest for the elderly and if like some of the elderly population who have trouble chewing and swallowing these foods are easily pureed.

Health Benefits for the Elderly

The elderly can suffer from all types of maladies ranging from hypertension, cardiac disease, diabetes, and osteoporosis. By making the switch to a vegetarian diet the risks of these ailments can be lessened somewhat. While it will not reverse years of damage caused by eating a diet high in fat it will help to lower their cholesterol and if they suffer from diabetes it can help bring their blood glucose levels into a more acceptable range. Like with most vegetarians, the elderly should probably take a vitamin B12 supplement to ensure they are receiving the recommended daily dosage.

Chapter 13

How to Properly Cook Vegetables Common in Vegetarian Cuisine

Broccoli

When you go to but broccoli at supermarket, look for it to have firm spears that are dark green with a high floret to stem ratio. What is great about broccoli is that it only takes a few minutes to cook, about four minutes in a microwave or it can be steamed in only five minutes. To prepare broccoli, trim the ends off each stalk a couple of inches below the florets. If you want to eat the stalk as well, it is recommended that you remove the outer layer with a vegetable peeler and then cut into desired size. The individual florets should then be trimmed from the head of the broccoli stalk. Broccoli is then ready to be cooked by whatever method you choose.

Eggplant

When you are choosing an eggplant at your local supermarket you want to choose one that is nice and smooth with a shiny skin, the eggplant should not have any soft spots and its skin should be wrinkle free. The best way to prepare eggplant is to cut into slices about a ½-inch thick, remove the skin lightly salt it and place the slices in a strainer and let it naturally drain for twenty to thirty minutes. You can then either cut the eggplant into the size that you want for your dish or keep the larger slices. Eggplant is a versatile vegetable and can be prepared in different ways. If you choose to fry the eggplant, only use a small amount of oil because eggplant can act like a sponge and soak up excess oil, frying eggplant usually takes about six to eight minutes depending on the thickness of eggplant. Eggplant is also great on a grill, before you place the eggplant on the grill lightly oil both sides, it is usually ready in about eight to ten minutes depending on the thickness of the eggplant. Eggplant is ready to eat when it has a tender texture.

Lentils

Lentils are a staple of most vegetarian diet and provide a good source of iron. You can easily find lentils pre-packaged at your local supermarket. When preparing lentils, it is good to remember that two cups will serve four people. The first thing that you want to do when getting ready to cook lentils is to wash them with cold water. Measure the number of lentils that you want to cook put it in a strainer and run cold water over them to ensure that they are free of any excess dirt or grit. When cooking lentils, you want to make sure that you use a pot that has some depth to it because lentils expand when they are cooked. The general rule for cooking lentils is to use two cups of water for every cup of lentils you want to cook. To spice up your lentil dish you can get creative and add spices, vegetables, or turn it into a hearty soup. Lentil recipes are only limited by your imagination, get a cookbook that specializes in vegetarian cuisine and you will be sure to find a plethora of recipes that include lentils.

Black Beans

Beans of all varieties play a large part in vegetarian cuisine. Black beans are a good source of protein, iron, thiamin, and folate. Before you start to cook black beans, it is best to inspect them for any dirt or grit and to make sure that there are not any beans that are cracked or are shrivelling. Black beans can take up to two hours to cook depending on their freshness; the fresher the beans are the less time is needed to cook them because they have more moisture inside of them. For the best results when cooking black beans, it is recommended that they be soaked in water overnight, when doing this it is best to have at least two inches of water covering the beans. When cooking black beans do not add anything to the pot such as salt or vegetables until the beans are almost finished cooking. Black beans are a wonderful addition to rice dishes and be sure to include your favourite vegetables for a wonderful meal.

Red Beans

Like black beans, red beans are also used quite a bit in vegetarian cooking. Red beans are a good source of protein, iron, folate, and dietary fiber. As with black beans, the first thing you should do before preparing red beans is to inspect them for dirt and grit. In addition if there are any beans that are discoloured discard them. If you choose to soak the beans overnight before cooking them it will decrease the cooking time, just be sure not to soak them for longer than twenty-four hours as this could lead to the beans beginning to ferment. When you are ready to start cooking, drain the beans from the water that they were soaking in a give them a good rinse. Change the water and cover the beans with water and bring them to a boil as soon as the water begins to boil reduce the heat and cover the pot. Let the beans simmer for one to three hours depending on the amount of beans you are cooking. You will know when the beans are done when they are soft and can be mashed easily. Red beans are great as a side dish by themselves or with rice.

Homemade Veggie burgers

Just because you have decided to become a vegetarian or have been one for as long as you can remember, it does not mean that you must give up on having a tasty burger. The great thing about veggie burgers is that there are all different kinds made from all types of vegetarian ingredients. For example, veggie burgers can be made from a combination of black beans and potatoes. To make these great tasting veggie burgers you will need one cup of canned black beans, ½ an onion, three medium sized potatoes, two scallions, and ½ cup of corn. To prepare the ingredients, you will want to dice the onion, grate the potatoes, and chop scallions. Then mash the black beans and then add the other ingredients mixing them well together. Then shape them into patties just like regular hamburgers add a couple of tablespoons of oil to the pan and cook about four minutes on each side. To add to the veggie burger top it with fresh avocado, tomatoes, or another of your favourite fresh vegetables.

Zucchini

When you are inspecting zucchini at supermarket you what to make sure that it does not have any soft spots or any breaks in its skin. Zucchini is favoured by vegetarians because it is a great source of vitamin C and is low in saturated fat and cholesterol. Moreover, zucchini is a versatile vegetable than can be cooked and served in numerous ways. You can cut it into slices approximately a ⅓ inch thick brush with oil and cook on the grill for about three to four minutes each side. It can be roasted in the oven at the same size as on the grill at five hundred degrees for approximately ten minutes with it being turned over once halfway through. One of the most famous dishes that zucchini is a part off is ratatouille.

To prepare ratatouille, you will need two eggplants peeled and cut into approximately one-inch cubes sprinkle with salt and place in a strainer and let it drain for two to three hours. Then cut two large zucchinis into the same sized cubes toss the eggplant, zucchini cubes together with a couple of tablespoons of oil place in a baking pan into oven that has been preheated to five hundred degrees. Roast eggplant and zucchini mixture for about forty minutes or until they are tender and brown. When the mixture is almost done, in a large pot heat a couple of tablespoons of oil and add one onion that has been chopped and sauté until it starts to soften and brown. Then add a couple of cloves of minced garlic along with two tomatoes that have been chopped and cook for an additional five minutes and finally add the eggplant and zucchini mixture and cook for five more minutes.

Tofu

Tofu is a staple of many vegetarian diets. Tofu is made by making curd from soymilk instead of milk from cows. Soybeans are an important part of a vegetarian's diet because it has all eight essential amino acids. Although tofu is relatively new in western culture it has been used in China for over a thousand years. You will be able to find tofu in the refrigerated section of your local supermarket and it comes in different varieties. You will be able to choose from extra firm, firm, soft, and silken. It is best to stick with the type of texture of tofu of whatever recipe you are following calls for. The different types of tofu are used for different kinds of recipes. The firm and extra firm types of tofu are good to use on the grill or in Chinese stir fry. Vegetarians like to use the soft variety as a substitute for cheese. The silken variety is used to add protein to pasta sauce, smoothies, and soups.

Cauliflower

When picking out cauliflower at your local supermarket you want to make sure that the head of the cauliflower is tight, white, or purple in colour without any brown or yellow spots.

Cauliflower is popular with vegetarians due to it being a good source of vitamin C, with one serving of cauliflower you can get seventy-seven percent of the recommended daily allowance.

Cauliflower, like many vegetables can be prepared in many ways from steaming, braising, and roasting. One way that cauliflower is now being used by vegetarians is as a puree. This is used to replace the starch of potatoes and can add a nice alternative and add that little something extra to your meal.

Zucchini Pie

Ingredients

- ❖ 1 1/2 cups grated zucchini

- ❖ 3/4 cup buttermilk baking mix

- ❖ 1 tomato, chopped

- ❖ 1/2 cup fresh corn kernels

- ❖ 1/2 cup diced onion

- ❖ 3/4 cup shredded Cheddar cheese

- ❖ 2 eggs, beaten

Directions

1. Preheat oven to 350 degrees F (175 degrees C).

2. Lightly butter one 9 inch pie plate.

3. In a medium bowl mix zucchini, buttermilk baking mix, tomato, corn, onion, cheese and eggs together.

4. Bake at 350 degrees F (175 degrees C) for 45 minutes.

Do not cover the dish while it is cooking. Serve warm.

Servings Per Recipe: 6

Whole Wheat Pasta with Cucumber and Spicy Peanut Sauce

Ingredients:

- ❖ 3/4 cup creamy peanut butter

- ❖ 3 tablespoons soy sauce

- ❖ 3 tablespoons lemon juice

- ❖ 2 garlic cloves, minced

- ❖ 1 teaspoon dried hot red pepper flakes

- ❖ 1 teaspoon sugar

- ❖ 1 cup hot water

- ❖ 20 ounces whole wheat pasta

- ❖ 2 cucumbers, peeled, seeded and cut diagonally into 1/8-inch slices

- ❖ 1 cup thinly sliced scallions

- ❖ 1 cup red peppers, thinly sliced and 1 inch in length

- ❖ salt and pepper to taste

Directions:

- ❖ In a blender combine the peanut butter, soy sauce, lemon juice, garlic,

- ❖ red pepper flakes, sugar and hot water until smooth. In a pot of boiling

- ❖ salted water, boil the pasta until just tender; transfer to colander and

- ❖ rinse briefly under cold water. Drain the pasta noodles well. In a large bowl,

- ❖ toss noodles with peanut sauce, cucumbers, scallions and red peppers.

- ❖ Add salt and pepper to taste. Serve immediately at room temperature.

Makes 8 servings.

Vietnamese Rice-Noodle Salad

Ingredients:

- ❖ 5 cloves garlic

- ❖ 1 cup loosely packed chopped cilantro

- ❖ 1/2 jalapeno pepper, seeded and minced

- ❖ 3 tablespoons white sugar

- ❖ 1/4 cup fresh lime juice

- ❖ 3 tablespoons vegetarian fish sauce, or 1 teaspoon salt

- ❖ 1 (12 ounce) package rice vermicelli

- ❖ 2 carrots, julienned

- ❖ 1 cucumber, halved lengthwise and chopped

- ❖ 1/4 cup coarsley chopped fresh mint

- ❖ 4 leaves napa cabbage

- ❖ 1/4 cup unsalted peanuts

- ❖ 4 sprigs fresh mint

Directions:

1. Mince the garlic with the cilantro and the hot pepper. Transfer the mixture to a bowl, add the lime juice, fish sauce or salt and sugar; stir well. Let the sauce sit for 5 minutes.

2. Bring a large pot of salted water to a boil. Add the rice noodles; boil them for 2 minutes. Drain well. Rinse the noodles with cold water until they have cooled. Let them drain again.

3. Combine the sauce, noodles, carrots, cucumber, mint and Napa cabbage in a large serving bowl. Toss well and serve the salad garnished with the peanuts and mint sprigs.

Veggies and Dip

Ingredients:

- ❖ 2 cups sour cream

- ❖ 1/2cup grated Parmesan cheese

- ❖ 1/2 tsp garlic powder

- ❖ 1/2 tsp celery salt assorted raw vegetables, scrubbed and cut into bite-sized pieces

Directions:

Mix first four ingredients well with sppon and refrigerate for at least one hour before serving.

19 g carbohydrates for entire recipe of dip.

Veggie Pot Pie

Prep Time: approx. 30 Minutes

Cook Time: approx. 1 Hour

Ingredients

- ❖ 2 tablespoons olive oil

- ❖ 1 onion, chopped

- ❖ 8 ounces mushrooms

- ❖ 1 clove garlic, minced

- ❖ 2 large carrots, diced

- ❖ 2 potatoes, peeled and diced

- ❖ 2 stalks celery, sliced 1/4 inch wide

- ❖ 1 teaspoon kosher salt

- ❖ 1 teaspoon ground black pepper

- ❖ 2 cups cauliflower florets

- ❖ 1 cup fresh green beans, snapped in 1/2-inch pieces

- ❖ 3 cups vegetable broth

- ❖ 2 tablespoons cornstarch

- ❖ 2 tablespoons soy sauce

- ❖ 1 recipe pastry for a 9-inch single crust pie

Directions

1. Preheat oven to 425 degrees F (220 degrees C).

2. Heat oil in a large skillet or saucepan. Add the onions, mushrooms, and garlic; saute briefly. Mix in the carrots, potatoes and celery. Sprinkle with salt and pepper; stir well.

3. Mix in the cauliflower, green beans and vegetable broth. Bring to a boil then turn heat down to a simmer and cook until vegetables are barely tender, about 5 minutes.

4. In a small bowl mix corn-starch, soy sauce, and 1/4 cup water until corn-starch is completely dissolved. Add this mixture to the pan of vegetables and stir until sauce thickens, about 3 minutes.

5. Press the crust into an 11x7 inch baking dish. Pour the filling into the crust and cover the pie filling with the top crust.

6. Bake for 30 minutes or until the crust is brown.

Servings Per Recipe: 6

Veggie Foils

Ingredients

- ❖ 3 white onions, sliced to 1/4-inch thickness

- ❖ 9 frozen small corn cobs

- ❖ 1/2 pound snow peas

- ❖ 3 tablespoons butter

- ❖ seasoning salt to taste

- ❖ 2 cubes ice

Directions

1. Lightly oil grill and preheat to high.

2. Place onion slices on a large sheet of aluminium foil; bring up edges of foil a bit to form a foil 'package'. Add corn and snow peas to onions. Place butter or margarine on top, spread out. Season with seasoned salt to taste, then lay ice cubes on top of the whole thing. Seal well in a foil 'packet'.

3. Place foil packet on top shelf of preheated grill while cooking your favourite meats; grill until corn is firm but tender.

Open foil packet and serve!

Vegetarian Link Gravy

Vegetarian sausage links can be bought at many supermarkets, experiment with the different brands and choose your favourited for this delicious gravy. If you would like a thicker gravy dissolve 1 tablespoon of corn-starch in 1 tablespoon warm water and mix into the gravy just before bringing it to a boil.

Ingredients

- ❖ 6 links vegetarian sausage

- ❖ 3 tablespoons olive oil

- ❖ 1 cup vegetable broth

- ❖ 1/8 cup all-purpose flour

- ❖ 1 teaspoon salt

- ❖ freshly ground black pepper

- ❖ 1/4 teaspoon dried sage

Directions

1. Place the vegetarian link or patties and 1 tablespoon oil in a large frying pan, fry the links until done.

2. Break the links into small pieces. Add the remaining oil and flour to a small pot. Mix the flour with the oil over medium low heat until a rue is formed. Slowly add the vegetable broth, mixing well.

3. Add the salt, pepper, sage and cooked sausage pieces. Bring mixture to a boil.

Makes 1 cup

Vegetarian Lasagna

Serving Size: 8

- ❖ Lasagna Noodles

- ❖ 10 ounce Pk frozen chopped Broccoli

- ❖ 14 1/2 ounce Can Tomatoes

- ❖ 15 ounce Can Tomato Sauce

- ❖ 1 cup Chopped Celery

- ❖ 1 cup Chopped Onion

- ❖ 1 cup Chopped Grn/Sweet Red Pepper

- ❖ 1 1/2 teaspoon Dried Basil crushed *

- ❖ Bay leaves

- ❖ Clove garlic minnced

- ❖ Beaten Egg

- ❖ 2 cup Lo-fat Ricotta or Cottage Ch

- ❖ 1/4 cup Grated Parmesan Cheese

- ❖ 1 cup Shredded Mozzarella Cheese

Directions:

Cook noodles and broccoli separately according to their package directions; drain well. Set aside.

For sauce, cut up canned tomatoes. In a large saucepan stir together undrained tomatoes, tomato sauce, celery, green or sweet red pepper, basil, bay leaves, and garlic. Bring to boiling; reduce heat. Simmer, uncover, 20-25 minutes or till sauce is thick, stirring occasionally.

Remove bay leaves. Meanwhile, in a bowl stir together egg, ricotta cheese, parmesan cheese, and 1/4 t pepper. Stir in broccoli.

Spread about 1/2 cup of the sauce in a 13x9x2" baking dish. Top with half the noodles, half of the broccoli mixture, and half of the remaining sauce.

Repeat layers, ending with the sauce.

Bake, uncovered, in a 350 deg F oven for 25 minutes; sprinkle with Mozzarella.

Bake 5 minutes more or till heated through. Let stand 10 minutes before serving.

Tzatziki

Prep Time: approx. 15 Minutes

This yogurt, cucumber, and garlic dip is a wonderful, cool companion dish - great for summer!

Ingredients

- ❖ 2 cucumbers - peeled, seeded, and quartered

- ❖ 1 tablespoon kosher salt

- ❖ 4 cloves garlic, minced

- ❖ 1 tablespoon lemon juice

- ❖ 1 1/2 cups plain yogurt

- ❖ 1 teaspoon distilled white vinegar

- ❖ 1/4 cup olive oil

Directions

1. Place quartered cucumbers in a small colander, sprinkle evenly with salt. Allow to drain 30 minutes. Pat dry with paper towels and chop coarsely in food processor. Drain cucumber in colander for an additional 30 minutes.

2. Place cucumber in food processor with garlic, lemon juice, yogurt, and vinegar. Blend well. Adjust vinegar and salt to taste. Pour in olive oil, blend until ingredients are well combined. Refrigerate until ready to serve.

Summer Pasta

Prep Time: approx. 10 Minutes

Cook Time: approx. 5 Minutes / Makes 6 servings

Ingredients

- ❖ 1 (16 ounce) package linguini pasta

- ❖ 6 Roma tomatoes

- ❖ 1 pound shredded mozzarella cheese

- ❖ 1/3 cup chopped fresh basil

- ❖ 6 cloves garlic, minced

- ❖ 1/2 cup olive oil, 1/2 teaspoon garlic salt

- ❖ ground black pepper to taste

Directions

1. Combine tomatoes, cheese, basil, garlic, olive oil, garlic salt, and black pepper in medium bowl. Set aside.

2. Meanwhile, cook pasta according to package directions. Drain pasta, and transfer to a serving bowl.

   Toss with tomato mixture. Serve.

Chapter 14

Do not be Afraid of New Things

As you have read, being or becoming a vegetarian is something that is never to late in life to do. The health benefits that you will get from switching from being an omnivore to a vegetarian are almost countless. If you are suffering from hypertension, cardiovascular disease, or diabetes.

Checklist

What Do Fruits and Vegetables Contain:

Vitamins – organic compounds that provide a range of roles in the human body.

Minerals – Metal, stone, and other inorganic compounds that form many of the structures in the human body.

Essential amino acids – The building blocks of protein that help form muscle, skin, brain tissue and more.

Essential fatty acids – Crucial for absorption of nutrients, formation of hormones, and more.

Fiber – Improves digestion, helps support a healthy gut flora.

Some Beneficial Minerals:

Calcium – Used to build bones and connective tissues. Used in the communication between cells.

Magnesium – Builds bones, in combination with calcium. Also increases testosterone production.

Zinc – Supports a stronger sense of smell, helps support testosterone in combination with magnesium. Important for brain health.

Potassium – An electrolyte that can prevent cramping.

Iron – Used to create haemoglobin. These are the red cells that carry blood and therefore oxygen around the body.

Some Beneficial Vitamins:

Vitamin C – Supports the immune system. Used to make the feel-good hormone serotonin.

Vitamin D – EVEN better than vitamin C for helping to fight colds. Regulates the production of crucial hormones like testosterone.

Vitamin A – Important for the skin, and eyes. Turns out it might also have a big role to play in brain health.

Vitamin B Complex – Among other things, helps the body to extract energy from carbs.

Other Useful Nutrients Found in Fruits and Vegetables:

Omega 3 fatty acid – One of the most important nutrients of all. Helps to boost brain function, fight inflammation, and more.

Lutein – Related to vitamin A. Helps to increase energy efficiency.

Polyphenols – Plant compounds that have many very beneficial effects in the body, many of which we still do not realize!

Antioxidants – Fight cancer.

Some Examples of Highly Beneficial Fruits and Vegetables

Garlic – Kills unwanted bacteria. Widens blood vessels. Aids digestion.

Beets – Used by athletes to improve their performance.

Mushrooms – Packed with lean protein and one of the only food sources of vitamin D.

Cherries – Help us sleep thanks to the content of melatonin.

Bananas – Rich in potassium to help prevent cramps, boost mood, and more.

Apples – High in vitamin C to strengthen the immune system. Also high in epicatechin, which can aid muscle growth.

Celery – The high-water content makes them hydrated, but they also contain fiber. Extremely low calorie and great for dieting.

Avocado – Extremely popular for those looking to follow a low carb diet. Also rich in omega 3 and more.

Red grapes – High in resveratrol, which may help us to live longer!

Benefits of Getting More Fruits and Vegetables:

More energy – wake up feeling great and last all day!

Better mood – more serotonin means you are less grumpy and less likely to feel sad.

Improved cognitive performance – say goodbye to brain fog, lack of focus, poor memory.

Better immune system to prevent yourself from getting colds and flus.

Fight cancer and aging by combating antioxidants.

Better body composition – lose weight and build muscle by supporting your metabolism.

Combat a host of specific illnesses and diseases.

Improve your microbiome and boost your gut health.

Risks of Too Much

Too much fruit can damage your teeth. Too much of either can lead to weight gain. Remember that even healthy foods still do contain calories!

While rare, it is possible to overdose on certain nutrients that are fat soluble.

How to get more fruits and vegetables

Use frozen packs and then break bits off into your cooking.

Used tinned. Cook meals like bolognaise and hot pots that allow you to throw lots of ingredients in. Cook more than you need and then freeze extra in individual pots to bring out as needed.

Get dried fruit – or dry your own!

Grow your own vegetables.

Diet mistakes:

When it comes to your diet, one SIMPLE change you can make to be FAR healthier and slimmer, is to cut out all "empty calories", all highly processed foods. An empty calorie is simply any food that is high in calories but that does not provide much in the way of nutrition as a result. This often means things like hot dogs, chocolate, chips. Fruits and vegetables offer precise opposite proposition. Consuming a multivitamin does not work as well. However, it can be somewhat useful as a backup.

Being a vegetarian can help you battle back against these maladies and can perhaps give you a better quality of life.

Being a vegetarian does not have to mean that your food must be bland and boring. Today more and more recipes are coming out that makes vegetarian cuisine fresh, vibrant, and exciting. The days of being a vegetarian and sitting down to a salad and a bowl of rice is no longer necessary as you have read. When you have made the decision to become a vegetarian go to your local bookstore and get several vegetarian cookbooks and take the time to experiment with all the recipes so you learn what you like and what you would rather not eat.

Remember, the vegetarian lifestyle has been around for thousands of years, so there must be something to it, otherwise it would have been long gone by now. Whether it came about through religion or out of necessity is not as important as the benefits that it brings to those who choose to live a vegetarian lifestyle. That is not to mention it helps people live in harmony with animals and the nature that surrounds us and not being a part of the unnecessary slaughter of livestock and poultry can help us live with a clearer conscious.

CPSIA information can be obtained
at www.ICGtesting.com
Printed in the USA
BVHW041517190321
602997BV00010B/615